APPLE CIDER
VINEGAR

Publications International, Ltd.

Note: The editors of Publications International, Ltd., nor the authors, consultants,
editors, or publisher take responsibility for any possible consequence from any
treatment, procedure, exercise, dietary modification, action, or application of
medication or preparation by any person reading or following the information in this
book. The publication of this book does not constitute the practice of medicine,
and this book does not attempt to replace your physician or your pharmacist.
Before undertaking any course of treatment, the authors, consultants, editors, and
publisher advise the reader to check with a physician or other health care provider.

CONTENTS

INTRODUCTION

If you were told that there were a new product on the market that could act as a general remedy and tonic, soothe skin ailments, condition your hair, clean your household, and add flavor to meals, you'd probably be skeptical. How could one substance do all those things? But age-old vinegar serves all those purposes.

There seems hardly an ailment that vinegar has not been touted to cure at some point in history. And while science has yet to prove the effectiveness of many of these folk cures, scores of people still praise and value vinegar as a healthful and healing food. In this book, we'll take a look at the history of vinegar, examine the healing claims made for it, and discuss how you can use vinegar in your life.

JUST WHAT IS VINEGAR?

Vinegar is a dilute solution of acetic acid that results from a two-step fermentation process. The first step is the fermentation of sugar into alcohol, usually by yeast. Any natural source of sugar can be used. For example, the sugar may be derived from the juice, or cider, of fruit (such as grapes, apples, raisins, or even coconuts); from a grain (such as barley or rice); from honey, molasses, or sugar cane; or even, in the case of certain distilled vinegars, from the cellulose in wood (such as beech).

What you have at the end of this first phase, then, is an alcohol-containing liquid, such as wine (from grapes), beer (from barley), hard cider (from apples), or another fermented liquid. The alcoholic liquid used to create a vinegar is generally reflected in the vinegar's name—for example, red wine vinegar, white wine vinegar, malt vinegar, or cider vinegar.

In the second phase of the vinegar-production process, certain naturally occurring bacteria known as acetobacters combine the alcohol-containing liquid with oxygen to form the acetic-acid solution we call vinegar. Acetic acid is what gives vinegar its sour taste. Although time-consuming, this second phase of the process will happen without human intervention if the alcoholic liquid is exposed to oxygen long enough.

ALL ABOUT ACIDITY

The U.S. Food and Drug Administration requires that vinegar contain a minimum of 4 percent acetic acid. White vinegar is typically 5 percent acetic acid, and cider and wine vinegars are a bit more acidic, usually between 5 percent and 6 percent.

A little acidity goes a long way—acetic acid is corrosive and can destroy living tissues when concentrated. An acetic acid level of 11 percent or more can burn the skin. And according to the Consumer Product Safety Commission, an "acetic acid preparation containing free or chemically unneutralized acetic acid in a concentration of 20 percent or more" is considered poison. In fact, a 20 percent acetic acid concentration is sometimes used as an herbicide to kill garden weeds.

THE HISTORY OF VINEGAR

The first vinegar was the result of an ancient, serendipitous, accident. Once upon a time, a keg of wine (presumably a poorly sealed one that allowed oxygen in) was stored too long, and when the would-be drinkers opened it, they found a sour liquid instead of wine. The name "vinegar" is derived from the French words for "sour wine."

Fortunately, our resourceful ancestors found ways to use the "bad" wine. They put it to work as a cure-all, a food preservative, and later, a flavor enhancer. It wasn't long before they figured out how to make vinegar on purpose, and producing it then became one of the world's earliest commercial industries.

Scientists believe wine originated during the Neolithic period (approximately 8500 B.C. to 4000 B.C., when humans first began farming and crafting stone tools) in Egypt and the Middle East. Large pottery jugs dating back to 6000 B .C. that were unearthed in archaeological digs possessed a strange yellow residue. Chemical analysis revealed the residue contained calcium tartrate, which is formed from tartaric acid, a substance that occurs naturally in large amounts only in grapes. So the traces strongly suggest the jugs were used to make or hold wine.

Considering the slow grape-pressing methods used at that time and the heat of the desert environment, grape juice would likely have fermented into wine quite quickly. Likewise, the wine would have turned to vinegar rapidly, if conditions were right.

So how did these ancient people—who had only recently (in evolutionary terms) begun planting their own food and fashioning tools—manage to understand and control fermentation enough to prevent all their wine from turning to vinegar before they could drink it? Based on evidence found in archaeological excavations, scientists believe that the first winemakers used jars with clay stoppers that helped control the fermentation process.

A complete analysis of the residue left in those ancient wine jugs also showed the presence of terebinth tree resin, which acts as a natural preservative and therefore would have helped slow the transformation of wine into vinegar. In Neolithic times, terebinth trees grew in the same area as grapes, and their berries and resin were harvested at the same time of year. So it's quite plausible that some of the berries or resins may have inadvertently become mixed with the grape harvest. Still unclear is whether the ancient winemakers ever made the connection between the resins and the delayed conversion of wine into vinegar and began purposely adding the tree berries to their wine.

TYPES OF VINEGAR

You might be surprised to learn that there are dozens of types of vinegar. The most common vinegars found in American kitchens are white distilled and apple cider, but the more adventurous may also use red wine vinegar, white wine vinegar, rice vinegar, or gourmet varieties, such as 25-year-old balsamic vinegar or rich black fig vinegar.

Vinegars can be made from many different foods that add their own tastes to the final products, but additional ingredients, such as herbs, spices, or fruits, can be added for further flavor enhancement.

Vinegar is great for a healthy, light style of cooking. The tangy taste often reduces the need for salt, especially in soups and bean dishes. It can also cut the fat in a recipe because it balances flavors without requiring the addition of as much cream, butter, or oil. Vinegar flavors range from mild to bold, so you're sure to find one with the taste you want. A brief look at some of the various vinegars available may help you choose a new one for your culinary escapades.

WHITE VINEGAR

This clear variety is the most common type of vinegar in American households. It is made either from grain-based ethanol or laboratory-produced acetic acid and then diluted with water. Its flavor is a bit too harsh for most cooking uses, but it is good for pickling and performing many cleaning jobs around the house. For more about cleaning, see page 60.

APPLE CIDER VINEGAR

Apple cider vinegar is the second-most-common type of vinegar in the United States. This light-tan vinegar made from apple cider adds a tart and subtle fruity flavor to your cooking. Along with its health uses, apple cider vinegar is best for salads, dressings, marinades, condiments, and most general vinegar needs.

WINE VINEGAR

This flavorful type of vinegar is made from a blend of either red wines or white wines and is common in Europe, especially Germany. Creative cooks often infuse wine vinegars with extra flavor by tucking in a few sprigs of well-washed fresh herbs, dried herbs, or fresh berries. You might find sherry

vinegar on the shelf next to the wine vinegars. This variety is made from sherry wine and is usually imported from Spain. Champagne vinegar (yes, made from the bubbly stuff) is a specialty vinegar and is quite expensive.

Wine vinegar excels at bringing out the sweetness of fruit, melon, and berries and adds a flavorful punch to fresh salsa.

BALSAMIC VINEGAR

There are two types of this popular and delicious vinegar, traditional and commercial. A quasi-governmental body in Modena, Italy (balsamic vinegar's birthplace), regulates the production of traditional balsamic vinegar. Traditional balsamic vinegars are artisanal foods, similar to great wines, with long histories and well-developed customs for their production. What you're more likely to find in most American grocery stores is the commercial type of balsamic vinegar. Some is made in Modena, but not by traditional methods. In fact, some balsamic vinegar isn't even made in Italy.

Whether you're lucky enough to get your hands on the traditional variety or you're using commercial-grade balsamic, the taste of this fine vinegar is like no other. Its sweet and sour notes are in perfect proportion. Balsamic's flavor is so intricate that it brings out the best in salty foods such as goat cheese, astringent foods such as spinach, and sweet foods such as strawberries.

RICE VINEGAR

Clear or very pale yellow, rice vinegar originated in Japan, where it is essential to sushi preparation. Rice vinegar is made from the sugars found in rice, and the aged, filtered final product has a mild, clean, and delicate flavor that is an excellent complement to ginger or cloves, sometimes with the addition of sugar.

Rice vinegar is popular in Asian cooking and is great sprinkled on salads and stir-fry dishes. Its gentle flavor is perfect for fruits and tender vegetables, too. Many cooks choose white rice vinegar for their recipes because it does not change the color of the food to which it is added. Red rice vinegar is good for soups and noodle dishes, and black rice vinegar works as a dipping sauce and in braised dishes.

MALT VINEGAR

This dark-brown vinegar, a favorite in Britain, is reminiscent of deep-brown ale. Many people prefer malt vinegar for pickling and as an accompaniment to fish and chips. It is also used as the basic type of cooking vinegar in Britain.

CANE VINEGAR

This type of vinegar is produced from the sugar cane and is used mainly in the Philippines. It is often light yellow and has a flavor profile similar to rice vinegar. Contrary to what you might think, cane vinegar is not any sweeter than other vinegars.

BEER VINEGAR

Beer vinegar has an appealing light-golden color and, as you might guess, is popular in Germany, Austria, Bavaria, and the Netherlands. It is made from beer, and its flavor depends on the brew from which it was made.

COCONUT VINEGAR

If you can't get your Asian recipes to taste "just right," it might be because you don't have coconut vinegar—a white vinegar with a sharp, acidic, slightly yeasty taste. This staple of Southeast Asian cooking is made from the sap of the coconut palm and is especially important to Thai and Indian dishes.

RAISIN VINEGAR

This slightly cloudy, brown vinegar is traditionally produced in Turkey and used in Middle Eastern cuisines. Try infusing it with a little cinnamon to bolster its mild flavor. Salad dressings made with raisin vinegar will add an unconventional taste to your greens.

A LONG MEDICINAL HISTORY

The use of vinegar as medicine probably started soon after it was discovered.

- Its healing virtues are extolled in records of the Babylonians.

- The great Greek physician Hippocrates reportedly used it as an antibiotic.

- Ancient Greek doctors poured vinegar into wounds and over dressings as a disinfectant, and they gave concoctions of honey and vinegar to patients recovering from illness.

- In Asia, early samurai warriors believed vinegar to be a tonic that would increase their strength and vitality.

- Vinegar has continued to be used as a medicine in more recent times. During the Civil War and World War I, for example, military medics used vinegar to treat wounds.

- Folk traditions around the world still espouse vinegar for a wide variety of ailments. Natural-healing enthusiasts and vinegar fans continue to honor and use many of those folk remedies.

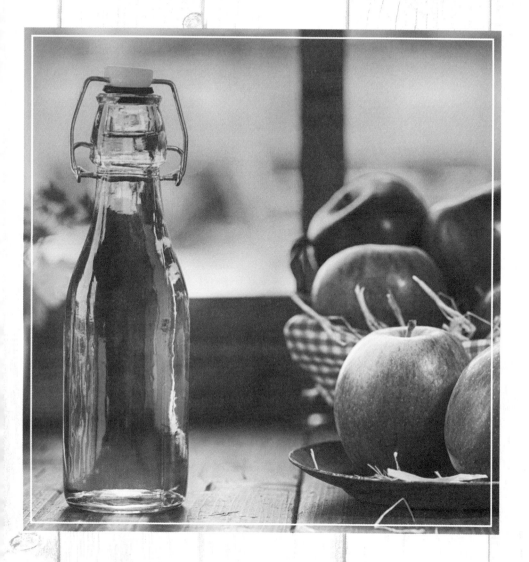

Vinegar's potential for treating or preventing major medical problems is of interest to almost everyone. But apple cider vinegar in particular has also has been cherished as a home remedy for some common minor ailments for centuries. Although they're not life-or-death issues, these minor health problems can be uncomfortable, and there is often little modern medicine can offer in the way of a cure. So you may want to give vinegar a shot to determine for yourself if it can help. (It's always best when trying any remedy for the first time to run it past your doctor to be sure there is no reason you should not try it.)

A GENERAL TONIC

One "recipe" for remaining healthy and alert well into the golden years combines good nutrition with an unusual beverage. Maintain a well-balanced diet, and drink a glass of water mixed with 1 teaspoon honey and 1 teaspoon apple cider vinegar at each of your 3 meals a day.

STOMACH AND BLADDER

To settle **minor stomach upset**, try a simple cider vinegar tonic with a meal. Drinking a mixture of a spoonful of vinegar in a glass of water is said to improve digestion and ease minor stomach upset by stimulating your digestive juices.

Morning sickness varies from woman to woman, even pregnancy to pregnancy. Many find this remedy helps to calm the stomach: Drink a glass of water mixed with 1 teaspoon apple cider vinegar first thing every morning.

Some **bladder infections** respond to this vinegar treatment: Three times a day, drink a glass of water mixed with 2 teaspoons apple cider vinegar. Be sure to consult your doctor first.

COLD, FLU, AND COUGH

Apple cider vinegar is an age-old treatment for symptoms of the common cold. For a **sore throat,** mix one teaspoon of apple cider vinegar into a glass of water; gargle with a mouthful of the solution and then swallow it, repeating until you've finished all the solution in the glass.

For a natural **cough syrup,** mix half a tablespoon apple cider vinegar with half a tablespoon honey and swallow.

Or mix 1/4 cup honey and apple cider vinegar; pour into a jar or bottle that can be tightly sealed. Shake well before each use. Take 1 tablespoon every 4 hours. If cough persists for more than a week, see a physician.

You can add a quarter-cup of apple cider vinegar to the recommended amount of water in your room vaporizer to help with congestion.

To alleviate a **sore throat** and also thin mucus, gargle with apple cider vinegar that has a little salt and ground black pepper added to it.

AN OLD-FASHIONED SORE-THROAT TONIC

The following came from a book of home remedies published more than 130 years ago. Some doctors still swear the tonic is surprisingly palatable and works wonders. (Do not give it or any other honey-containing food or beverage to children younger than two years of age. Honey can carry a bacterium that can cause a kind of food poisoning called infant botulism and may also cause allergic reactions in very young children.)

- One tablespoon honey, any kind
- One tablespoon vinegar, preferably apple-cider vinegar
- Eight ounces hot water

Mix all the ingredients together in a mug and sip slowly (but don't let it get cold). Use as often as desired.

TREATING MINOR SKIN AILMENTS

Relieve **itching or stinging from minor insect bites.** In the folk medicine of New England, rural Indiana, and parts of the Southwest, a vinegar wash is sometimes used for treating bites and stings. (However, if the person bitten has a known allergy to insect venom or begins to exhibit signs of a serious allergic reaction, such as widespread hives, swelling of the face or mouth, difficulty breathing, or loss of consciousness, skip the home remedies and seek immediate medical attention.) Dab the area with a cotton ball moistened with apple cider vinegar, avoiding surrounding healthy skin as much as possible. Then rinse. Or, use vinegar mixed with cornstarch to make a paste. Apply paste to a bee sting or bug bite and let dry.

To relieve **itchy skin**, add 1 cup apple cider vinegar to a bathtub of warm water. Soak in tub for at least 15 minutes.

Use your freezer to soothe and cool just about any kind of **skin itchiness**, be it from sunburn, a bug bite, or a rash. Fill each compartment of an empty, clean foam egg carton with apple cider vinegar; freeze. When the itch gets insane, pop out a vinegar cube and rub it over the spot.

One way to eliminate **athlete's foot** (or other fungal infections) is to create an environment that is inhospitable to the fungus that causes the condition. The Amish traditionally use a footbath of vinegar and water to discourage the growth of athlete's foot fungus. To try this remedy, mix one cup of vinegar into two quarts of water in a basin or pan. Soak your feet in this solution every night for 15 to 30 minutes, using a fresh solution each night. Or, if you prefer, mix up a solution using one cup of vinegar and one cup of water. Apply the solution to the affected parts of your feet with a cotton ball. Let your feet dry completely before putting on socks and/or shoes.

PSORIASIS

Psoriasis is a noncontagious, chronic skin condition that produces round, dry, scaly patches that are covered with white, gray, or silver-white scales. These patches are called plaques.

Although psoriasis is a mysterious condition (doctors aren't exactly sure what causes it or why it can be mild one day and serious the next), it is common. According to information from the National Institutes of Health, between 5.8 million and 7.5 million Americans have the disease. Psoriasis is also tough to treat because what works for one person may not work for another, and treatments that were once effective for an individual often become ineffective, and vice versa.

One solution that some people have found helpful to try is an apple cider vinegar dip. It's a great soak for affected fingernails and toenails; just pour some in a bowl or cup and dip your nails in for a few minutes. Some people have also had success applying it to plaques using cotton balls.

GENERAL SKIN CARE

Are your hands a mess from grease, gardening, or generally getting things done? **Clean very dirty hands** by scrubbing with cornmeal that has been moistened with a little bit of apple cider vinegar. Thoroughly scrub your hands—don't miss a grimy finger, knuckle, nail, or palm. Rinse well and dry; repeat if necessary. Your hands will be soft and smooth—and the dirt will be gone!

Vinegar mixed with onion juice may help reduce the appearance of age spots. Mix equal parts of onion juice and vinegar, and dab onto **age spots.** After several weeks of this routine, spots should lighten.

Apple cider vinegar is a great **aftershave** for men that will keep their skin soft and young looking. Keep a small bottle of it in the medicine cabinet, and splash on your face after shaving.

Make a **basic skin toner** using a mixture of equal parts apple cider vinegar or distilled white vinegar and water. Keep toner in a small spray bottle and apply after your usual wash.

FACIAL CARE

Control **oily skin** with a mixture of equal parts apple cider vinegar and cool water. The mixture works as an astringent. You can also freeze this solution into ice cubes and use it as a cooling facial treatment on a hot summer day.

Create your own **facial splash**. Boil 1 quart apple cider vinegar in microwave for 3 minutes in a large glass measuring cup. Remove and add herbs (lavender or rosemary are excellent). Pour into a sterilized bottle. Chill in refrigerator if desired.

Use a mixture of half vinegar, half water to **clean and tone your face**. Then rinse with vinegar diluted with water, and let your face air-dry to seal in moisture.

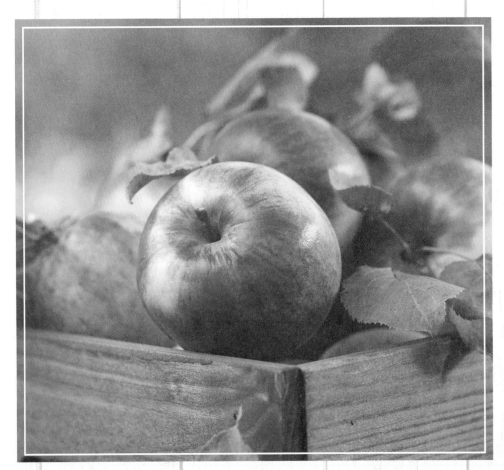

HAIR CARE

Vinegar is a great **hair conditioner** and can improve cleanliness and shine. For simple conditioning, just add one tablespoon vinegar to your hair as you rinse it.

Before shampooing, briefly soak hair in a small basin of water with 1/4 cup apple cider vinegar added. Repeat several times a week to help **control dandruff** and **remove buildup** from sprays, shampoos, and conditioners.

Use 1 tablespoon apple cider vinegar mixed with 1 gallon water as an after-shampoo rinse to **minimize gray** in your hair.

ACHES AND SORE MUSCLES

To relieve **achy muscles**, add 1 cup apple cider vinegar to a bathtub of warm water. Soak in tub for at least 15 minutes.

Another remedy for **sore muscles** is to boil 1 cup apple cider vinegar and add 1 teaspoon ground red pepper during boil. Cool this mixture, then apply it in a compress to sore area. Make sure pepper doesn't irritate the skin. The compress should make the area feel warm but not burning.

Try this liniment during a rubdown to relieve **achy muscles and arthritis pain**: Mix 1 cup apple cider vinegar, 1 cup extra virgin olive oil, and 2 egg whites. Massage into the painful parts; use a clean cotton cloth to wipe off any excess.

HICCUPS

Stop the **hiccups** with this old-time technique: Add 1 teaspoon apple cider vinegar to a glass of warm water. Sip very slowly until hiccups cease.

NOSEBLEEDS

Slow a **nosebleed** by soaking a cotton ball in diluted apple cider vinegar. Insert it gently into the bleeding nostril; hold your nose closed with your fingers. Breathe through your mouth for about 5 minutes. Carefully pull out the cotton. Repeat if your nose is still bleeding.

CURE-ALL FOR LONG TERM CONDITIONS?

The folk- and natural-healing claims made for vinegar through the ages have been plentiful and varied. Even in the current era of high-tech medicine, some proponents of natural healing still encourage traditional uses of vinegar. They have also added certain newly recognized or newly defined (within the past hundred years or so, that is) medical conditions to the list of health concerns for which they recommend vinegar.

Other present-day apple cider vinegar fans view it as an overall health-boosting, disease-fighting tonic and recommend mixing a teaspoon or tablespoon of cider vinegar with a glass of water and drinking it each morning or before meals.

Perhaps most amazingly, vinegar is heralded as a potential healer of many of today's most common serious ailments. Devotees believe vinegar can help prevent or heal heart disease, diabetes, obesity, cancer, aging-related ailments, and a host of other conditions. They say it is full of vitamins, minerals, fiber, enzymes, and pectin and often attribute vinegar's medicinal effects to the presence of these ingredients. The following are some of the specific claims made for apple cider vinegar:

It reduces blood cholesterol levels and heart-disease risk. Apple cider vinegar fans say it contains pectin, which attaches to cholesterol and carries it out of the body, thus decreasing the risk of heart disease. In addition, many vinegar proponents say it is high in potassium, and high-potassium foods play a role in reducing the risk of heart disease by helping to prevent or lower high blood pressure. Calcium is also an important nutrient for keeping blood pressure in check, and vinegar is sometimes promoted as having a high calcium content. Many also claim vinegar helps the body absorb this essential mineral from other foods in the diet.

It treats diabetes. Apple cider vinegar may help control blood sugar levels, which helps to ward off diabetes complications, such as nerve damage and blindness. It also might help prevent other serious health problems, such as heart disease, that often go hand-in-hand with diabetes.

It fights obesity and aids in weight loss. Some marketers proclaim that apple cider vinegar is high in fiber and therefore aids in weight loss. (Fiber provides bulk but is indigestible by the body, so foods high in fiber provide a feeling of fullness for fewer calories.) A daily dose is also said to control or minimize the appetite. (Ironically, some folk traditions advise taking apple cider vinegar before a meal for the opposite effect—to stimulate the appetite in people who have lost interest in eating.)

It prevents cancer and aging. Apple cider vinegar proponents declare it contains high levels of the antioxidant beta-carotene (a form of vitamin A) and therefore helps prevent cancer and the ill effects of aging. (Antioxidants help protect the body's cells against damage from unstable molecules called free radicals; free-radical damage has been linked to various conditions, including coronary heart disease, cancer, and the aging process.)

It prevents osteoporosis. Advocates say apple cider vinegar releases calcium and other minerals from the foods you eat so your body is better able to absorb and use them to strengthen bones. Vinegar allegedly allows the body to absorb one-third more calcium from green vegetables than it would without the aid of vinegar. Some fans also say apple cider vinegar is itself a great source of calcium.

Based on these claims, apple cider vinegar certainly seems to be a wonder food. And it's understandably tempting to want to believe that some food or drug or substance will make diabetes, obesity, cancer, and osteoporosis go away with little or no discomfort, effort, or risk.

However, as a wise consumer, you know that when something sounds too good to be true, it almost certainly is. So when it comes to your health—especially when you're dealing with such major medical conditions—it's important to take a step back and look carefully at the evidence.

A CLOSER LOOK AT THE CLAIMS

With such dramatic claims made for it, you would think that vinegar would be high on the lists of medical researchers searching for the next breakthrough. Yet in the past few decades, there has been very little research into the use of vinegar for therapeutic health purposes.

Granted, a lack of supporting scientific research is a common problem with many natural and alternative therapies. But even the National Center for Complementary and Alternative Medicine (NCCAM), a division of the U.S. government's National Institutes of Health that was created specifically to investigate natural or unconventional therapies that hold promise, has not published any studies about vinegar, despite the fact that there has been renewed interest in vinegar's healing benefits recently.

So without solid scientific studies, can we judge whether vinegar provides the kinds of dramatic benefits that its promoters and fans attribute to it? Not conclusively. But we can look at the claims and compare them to the little scientific knowledge we do have about vinegar.

Those who have faith in apple cider vinegar as a wide-ranging cure say its healing properties come from an abundance of nutrients that remain after apples are fermented to make apple cider vinegar. They contend that vinegar is rich in minerals and vitamins, including calcium, potassium, and beta-carotene; complex carbohydrates and fiber, including the soluble fiber pectin; amino acids (the building blocks of protein); beneficial enzymes; and acetic acid (which gives vinegar its taste).

These substances do play many important roles in health and healing, and some are even considered essential nutrients for human health. The problem is that standard nutritional analysis of vinegar, including apple cider vinegar, has not shown it to be a good source of most of these substances.

Take a look at the table on pages 34-35—it shows the results of a nutritional analysis of an apple compared with the nutritional breakdown of two different amounts of apple cider vinegar. One tablespoon of apple cider vinegar per day is the typical therapeutic dose recommended, so the nutrients found in this amount of the vinegar are shown in the second column of the table. Just to be sure that the small amount of vinegar in a tablespoon isn't the sole explanation for the apparent lack of nutrients, the table also includes the nutritional analysis of a larger amount (half a cup) of vinegar. You'll notice that even at that higher dose, vinegar does not appear to include significant amounts of most of the nutrients that are claimed to be the source of its medicinal value.

To put all this information into some context, the column at the far right in the table shows the daily amounts needed by a typical adult who consumes 2,000 calories per day. (Requirements haven't been established for some of the other substances that are often cited as contributing to vinegar's beneficial effects.)

As you can see, the one milligram of calcium in one tablespoon of apple cider vinegar does not come close to the 300 milligrams of calcium in eight ounces of milk, as some promoters of apple cider vinegar claim. In fact, it supplies only a tiny fraction of the 1,000 milligrams a typical adult needs in a day. Vinegar also contains little potassium.

In terms of pectin, the type of soluble fiber that is said to bind to cholesterol and help carry it out of the body, apple cider vinegar contains no measurable amounts of it or of any other type of fiber. So it would seem that pectin could not account for any cholesterol-binding activity that vinegar might be shown to have.

Do apple cider vinegar's secrets lie in the vitamins it contains? No. According to the USDA, apple cider vinegar contains no vitamin A, vitamin B 6 , vitamin C, vitamin E, vitamin K, thiamin, riboflavin, niacin, pantothenic acid, or folate.

What about some of the other health-boosting substances that are alleged to be in vinegar? According to detailed nutritional analyses, apple cider vinegar contains no significant amounts of amino acids. Nor does it contain ethyl alcohol, caffeine, theobromine, beta-carotene, alpha-carotene, beta-cryptoxanthin, lycopene, lutein, or zeaxanthin.

Nutrient	One medium apple, raw ($2^3/_4$ inch diameter)	1 Tbsp. apple cider vinegar	$^1/_2$ cup apple cider vinegar	Daily amount needed by avg. adult
Calories	72	3	25	2,000
Carbohydrate	19.06 g	0.14 g	1.11 g	130 g
Fat	0.23 g	0 g	0 g	65 g (max.)
Protein	0.36 g	0 g	0 g	46 g (women) 56 g (men)
Fiber	3.3 g	0 g	0 g	25 g (women) 38 g (men)
MINERALS				
Calcium	8 mg	1 mg	8 mg	1,000 mg
Iron	0.17 mg	0.03 mg	0.24 mg	18 mg (women) 8 g (men)

Nutrient	One medium apple, raw (2³/₄ inch diameter)	1 Tbsp. apple cider vinegar	¹/₂ cup apple cider vinegar	Daily amount needed by avg. adult
Magnesium	7 mg	1 mg	6 mg	320 g (women) 420 g (men)
Phosphorus	15 mg	1 mg	10 mg	700 mg
Potassium	148 mg	11 mg	87 mg	4,700 mg
Sodium	1 mg	1 mg	6 mg	1,500 mg
Zinc	0.06 mg	0.01 mg	0.05 mg	8 mg (women) 11mg (men)
Copper	0.037 mg	0.001 mg	0.01 mg	900 mcg
Manganese	0.048 mg	0.037 mg	0.298 mg	1.8 mg (women) 2.3 mg (men)
Selenium	0 mcg	0 mcg	0.1 mcg	55 mcg

HOW VINEGAR *CAN* HELP

So if vinegar doesn't actually contain all the substances that are supposed to account for its medicinal benefits, does that mean it has no healing powers? Hardly. As mentioned, so little research has been done on vinegar that we can't totally rule out many of the dramatic claims made it.

Although we know vinegar doesn't contain loads of nutrients traditionally associated with good health, it may well contain yet-to-be-identified phytochemicals (beneficial compounds in plants) that would account for some of the healing benefits that vinegar fans swear by. Scientists continue to discover such beneficial substances in all kinds of foods.

But beyond that possibility, there appear to be more tangible and realistic—albeit less sensational—ways that vinegar can help the body heal. Rather than being the dramatic blockbuster cure that we are endlessly (and fruitlessly) searching for, vinegar seems quite capable of playing myriad supporting roles—as part of an overall lifestyle approach—that can help us fight serious health conditions, such as osteoporosis, diabetes, and heart disease.

INCREASING CALCIUM ABSORPTION

If there is one thing vinegar fans, marketers, alternative therapists, and scientists alike can agree on, it's that vinegar is high in acetic acid. And acetic acid, like other acids, can increase the body's absorption of important minerals from the foods we eat. Therefore, including apple cider vinegar in meals or possibly even drinking a mild tonic of vinegar and water (up to a tablespoon of vinegar in a glass of water) just before or with meals might improve your body's ability to absorb the essential minerals locked in foods.

Vinegar may be especially useful to women, who generally have a hard time getting all the calcium their bodies need to keep bones strong and prevent the debilitating, bone-thinning disease osteoporosis. Although dietary calcium is most abundant in dairy products such as milk, many women (and men) suffer from a condition called lactose intolerance that makes it difficult or impossible for them to digest the sugar in milk. As a result, they may suffer uncomfortable gastrointestinal symptoms, such as cramping and diarrhea, when they consume dairy products. These women must often look elsewhere to fulfill their dietary calcium needs.

Dark, leafy greens are good sources of calcium, but some of these greens also contain compounds that inhibit calcium absorption. Fortunately for dairy-deprived women (and even those who do drink milk), a few splashes of vinegar or a tangy vinaigrette on their greens may very well allow them to absorb more valuable calcium.

CONTROLLING BLOOD SUGAR LEVELS

Vinegar has recently won attention for its potential to help people with type 2 diabetes get a better handle on their disease. Improved control could help them delay or prevent such complications as blindness, impotence, and a loss of feeling in the extremities that may necessitate amputation.

Also, because people with diabetes are at increased risk for other serious health problems, such as heart disease, improved control of their diabetes could potentially help to ward off these associated conditions, as well.

With type 2 diabetes, the body's cells become resistant to the action of the hormone insulin. The body normally releases insulin into the bloodstream in response to a meal. Insulin's job is to help the body's cells take in the glucose, or sugar, from the carbohydrates in food, so they can use it for energy.

But when the body's cells become insulin resistant, sugar from food begins to build up in the blood, even while the cells themselves are starving for it. (High levels of insulin tend to build up in the blood, too, because the body releases more and more insulin to try to transport the large amounts of sugar out of the bloodstream and into the cells.)

Over time, high levels of blood sugar can damage nerves throughout the body and otherwise cause irreversible harm. So one major goal of diabetes treatment is to normalize blood sugar levels and keep them in a healthier range as much as possible. And that's where vinegar appears to help.

It seems that vinegar may be able to inactivate some of the digestive enzymes that break the carbohydrates from food into sugar, thus slowing the absorption of sugar from a meal into the bloodstream. Slowing sugar absorption gives the insulin-resistant body more time to pull sugar out of the blood and thus helps prevent the blood sugar level from rising so high. Blunting the sudden jump in blood sugar that would usually occur after a meal also lessens the amount of insulin the body needs to release at one time to remove the sugar from the blood.

A study cited in 2004 in the American Diabetes Association's publication *Diabetes Care* indicates that vinegar holds real promise for helping people with diabetes. In the study, 21 people with either type 2 diabetes or insulin resistance (a prediabetic condition) and 8 control subjects were each given a solution containing five teaspoons of vinegar, five teaspoons of water, and one teaspoon of saccharin two minutes before ingesting a high-carbohydrate meal. The blood sugar and insulin levels of the participants were measured before the meal and 30 minutes and 60 minutes after the meal.

Vinegar increased overall insulin sensitivity 34 percent in the study participants who were insulin-resistant and 19 percent in those with type 2 diabetes. That means their bodies actually became more receptive to insulin, allowing the hormone to do its job of getting sugar out of the blood and into the cells. Both blood sugar and blood insulin levels were lower than usual in the insulin-resistant participants, which is more good news. Surprisingly, the control group (who had neither diabetes nor a prediabetic condition but were given the vinegar solution) also experienced a reduction in insulin levels in the blood. These findings are significant because, in addition to the nerve damage caused by perpetually elevated blood sugar levels, several chronic conditions, including heart disease, have been linked to excess insulin in the blood over prolonged periods of time.

More studies certainly need to be done to confirm the extent of vinegar's benefits for type 2 diabetes patients and those at risk of developing this increasingly common disease. But for now, people with type 2 diabetes might be wise to talk with their doctors or dietitians about consuming more vinegar.

REPLACING UNHEALTHY FATS AND SODIUM

There are some delicious varieties of vinegar available—and you're not limited to apple cider vinegar to get the benefits! Each bestows a different taste or character on foods. The diversity and intensity of flavor are key to one important healing role that vinegar can play. Whether you are trying to protect yourself from cardiovascular diseases, such as heart disease, high blood pressure, or stroke, or you have been diagnosed with one or more of these conditions and have been advised to clean up your diet, vinegar should become a regular cooking and dining companion.

That's because a tasty vinegar can often be used in place of sodium and/or ingredients high in saturated or trans fats to add flavor and excitement to a variety of dishes.

Saturated and trans fats have been shown to have a detrimental effect on blood cholesterol levels, and experts recommend that people who have or are at risk of developing high blood pressure cut back on the amount of sodium they consume. Using vinegar as a simple, flavorful substitute for these less healthful ingredients as often as possible can help people manage blood cholesterol and blood pressure levels and, in turn, help ward off heart disease and stroke.

The following suggestions will give you some sense of how vinegar can help you create and enjoy a diet that may lower your blood cholesterol and blood pressure and decrease your risks of heart disease and stroke:

- Make a vinegar-based coleslaw rather than a creamy, mayonnaise-based one. Because mayonnaise is made up almost completely of unhealthy fats and cholesterol, this easy switch can dramatically reduce the cholesterol and fat in this popular side dish.

- Enjoy healthier fish and chips. Instead of dipping fish in tartar sauce and drenching fries in salt and ketchup, splash them with a little malt vinegar. (Also consider baking the fish and the potatoes instead of frying them.) Because it contains mayonnaise, tartar sauce is high in unhealthy fats and cholesterol.

- Use vinegar-based salad dressings instead of creamy, mayonnaise-based dressings. Choose or make a flavorful herb salad dressing that contains mostly water, vinegar, and just a touch of oil to help it adhere to your salad veggies.

- Opt for vinegar instead of mayonnaise or other common, bad-fat-laden sandwich spreads to add flavor and moisture to sandwiches.

- When making a dish that contains beans, add a little vinegar near the end of cooking—it will dramatically decrease the amount of salt you'll need. It perks up the flavor of beans without raising your blood pressure.

- You can also use vinegar as a tangy marinade for tenderizing less-fatty cuts of meat. Choosing meat with less fat on the edges and less marbling within is one of the easiest ways to trim unhealthy fats from your diet. Unfortunately, meats that don't have as much marbling tend to be a little tougher. So vinegar can do double duty by adding a dash of zing as it tenderizes.

Vinegar loses some of its pungency when heated. If you want to enjoy vinegar's full tart taste, add it to a dish at the end of cooking. Also, after heating up leftovers, splash them with vinegar to perk up their flavors.

NEGAR

apple cider vinegar

Vinegar

ADDING EXCITEMENT TO A HEALTHY DIET

Some of our strongest natural weapons against cancer and aging are fruits and vegetables. The antioxidants and phytochemicals they contain seem to hold real promise in lowering our risk of many types of cancer. Their antioxidants also help to protect cells from the free-radical damage that is thought to underlie many of the changes we associate with aging. Protected cells don't wear out and need replacing as often as cells that aren't bathed in antioxidants. Scientists think this continual cell replacement may be at the root of aging.

It is recommended that the average person eat about two cups of fruit and two-and-a-half cups of vegetables every day. One way to add excitement and variety to all those vegetables is to use vinegar liberally as a seasoning.

- Rice vinegar and a little soy sauce give veggies an Asian flavor or can form the base of an Asian coleslaw.

- Red wine vinegar or white wine vinegar can turn boring vegetables into a quick-and-easy marinated-vegetable salad that's ready to be grabbed out of the refrigerator whenever hunger strikes. Just chop your favorite veggies, put them in a bowl with a marinade of vinegar, herbs, and a dash of olive oil, and let them sit for at least an hour. (You don't need much oil to make the marinade stick to the veggies, so go light, and be sure you choose olive oil.)

- Toss chopped vegetables in a vinegar-and-olive-oil salad dressing before loading them on skewers and putting them on the backyard grill. The aroma and flavor will actually have your family asking for seconds—of vegetables!

- After steaming vegetables, drizzle a little of your favorite vinegar over them instead of adding butter or salt. They'll taste so good, you may never get to the meat on your plate.

- When poaching fish, put a tablespoon of vinegar in the poaching water to keep the fish from falling apart. Vinegar helps the protein in the fish coagulate, and mushiness isn't a problem because fish is usually poached for less than 20 minutes.

- When a recipe calls for buttermilk and you have none, substitute plain milk and add a little apple cider vinegar. Use one tablespoon of vinegar per cup (eight ounces) of milk. Let stand 10 to 15 minutes at room temperature until it thickens, then use it in your recipe as you would buttermilk. Mild-flavored vinegars such as apple cider vinegar are best for this purpose.

- Cover peeled potatoes with water and a tablespoon or two of vinegar to keep them from browning.

- By enhancing the flavor of vegetables with vinegar, you and your family will be inclined to eat more of them. And that—many researchers and doctors would agree—will likely go a long way toward protecting your body's cells from the damage that can lead to cancer and other problems of aging.

REMOVING HARMFUL SUBSTANCES FROM PRODUCE

Some people are concerned that eating large amounts of fruits and vegetables may lead to an unhealthy consumption of pesticides and other farm-chemical residues. Vinegar can lend a hand here, too. Washing produce in a mixture of water and vinegar appears to help remove certain pesticides, according to the small amount of research that has been published. Vinegar also appears to be helpful in getting rid of harmful bacteria on fruits and vegetables.

To help remove potentially harmful residues, mix a solution of 10 percent vinegar to 90 percent water (for example, mix one cup of white vinegar in nine cups of water). Then, place produce in the vinegar solution, let it soak briefly, and then swish it around in the solution. Finally, rinse the produce thoroughly.

Do not use this process on tender, fragile fruits, such as berries, that might be damaged in the process or soak up too much vinegar through their porous skins. Some pesticide residues are trapped beneath the waxy coatings that are applied to certain vegetables to help them retain moisture. The vinegar solution probably won't wash those pesticides away, so peeling lightly may be a better option. Some research suggests that cooking further eliminates some pesticide residue.

ADDING FLAVOR, NOT CALORIES

Vinegar contains very few calories—only 25 in half a cup! Compare that to the nearly 800 calories you get in half a cup of mayonnaise, and you have a real fat-fighting food. So if you're looking to lose weight, using vinegar in place of mayonnaise whenever you can will help you make a serious dent in your calorie (and fat) intake.

Vinegar can also help you have your dessert and cut calories, too. Use a splash of balsamic vinegar to bring out the sweetness and flavor of strawberries without any added sugar. Try it on other fruits that you might sprinkle sugar on—you'll be pleasantly surprised at the difference a bit of balsamic vinegar can make. And for a real unexpected treat on a hot summer evening, drizzle balsamic vinegar—instead of high-fat, sugary caramel or chocolate sauce—on a dish of reduced-fat vanilla ice cream. Can't imagine that combination? Just try it.

VINEGAR AND GARLIC

Vinegar is good for you, and garlic is great. Why not combine the two and make pickled garlic? Simply peel some garlic cloves, cube them, and let them sit for 10 to 15 minutes to form allicin, a powerful sulfur-containing agent that helps protect your body's cells from damage. Then add the garlic to your favorite vinegar.

Vinegar helps garlic form healthful sulfur-containing compounds that are not otherwise formed in large amounts. The longer the garlic is in the vinegar, the more sulfur compounds it forms. Store your pickled garlic in the refrigerator and add it to salads and vegetable side dishes. What a delicious way to take your medicine—maybe a pickled clove a day will keep the doctor away.

SHOULD YOU SUPPLEMENT?

Some people believe in the healing power of apple cider vinegar but would rather take it in tablet form instead of using it as a daily tonic or adding it to food.

But like any shortcut on the road to better health, you can't be sure this one will get you to the goal you're aiming for.

Part of the reason for concern is that the U.S. Food and Drug Administration (FDA) does not regulate supplements, so you really can't be sure what you're getting. In a study reported in the July 2005 *Journal of the American Dietetic Association,* for example, researchers analyzed eight different brands of apple cider vinegar tablets. The analysis showed most had acetic acid levels different from those claimed on the label. How much of a problem is this? Well, it would be natural to think the more acetic acid the better. But in truth, at a level of 11 percent, acetic acid can cause burns to the skin. And at 20 percent, it is considered poisonous. Some of the analyzed supplements, however, claimed to contain a frightening 35 percent acetic acid! Fortunately for their users, none did. The acetic acid content actually ranged from 1.04 percent to 10.57 percent. Another reason to go natural: Several of the samples were contaminated with mold and/or yeast, including one that claimed to be yeast-free. In addition, because so little scientific research has been done to verify the healing claims made for vinegar—and the possible ingredients or actions that might be responsible—it's impossible to know if supplements would have the same effects as the real thing. Indeed, most of vinegar's benefits—at least the ones that rest on the most solid scientific grounds—are those based on its use as a substitute for unhealthy ingredients in the diet, a role that simply could not be played by a pill.

So at this time, it would seem you are almost certainly better off including more vinegar in your diet, taking advantage of its potential healing benefits as well as its phenomenal flavors, rather than spending more money on supplements that may not have any benefit and could even be dangerous.

PASTEURIZED FOR YOUR PROTECTION

Some apple cider vinegars proudly proclaim to be "raw, organic, and unpasteurized," but beware: Buying an unpasteurized product is risky business.

Most apple cider is made from apples that have fallen to the ground, and the bacterium *E. coli* can easily contaminate these fruits. If processors don't wash off this deadly bacterium before the apples are pressed, and the final product is not pasteurized, there is a risk of *E. coli* contamination, which can lead to severe health problems and even death.

Although most bacteria cannot survive in the acidic conditions of vinegar, the acidity of the unpasteurized product can weaken over time, thus allowing bacteria to grow—and making the product dangerous for you. To be on the safe side, be sure you always choose vinegars that have been prepared, pasteurized, and stored properly.

MAKE YOUR OWN APPLE CIDER VINEGAR

Perhaps reading about all the exciting uses of vinegar has whetted your appetite to make some of your own.

Experimenting with flavors can be fun, and it's especially rewarding to use your own vinegar in your favorite dishes or to give it as a gift.

You'll want to get exact directions from your local brewing supply store or university extension service. Be sure the directions you follow are tested and researched for safety to avoid food-borne illness. Take a look at this rundown of the general process to make apple cider vinegar to see if you're up to the task:

- Make apple cider by pressing clean, washed, ripe apples (fall apples have more sugar than early-season apples). Strain to make a clean juice and pour it into sterilized containers.

- Use yeast designed for brewing wine or beer (not baker's yeast) to ferment the fruit sugar into alcohol.

- Now let bacteria convert the alcohol to acetic acid. Leaving the fermenting liquid uncovered invites acid-making bacteria to take up residence. (You might, however, want to place some cheesecloth or a towel over your container's opening to prevent insects, dirt, or other nasty items from getting into the mixture.) Some vinegar brewers use a "mother of vinegar" (see the next page) as a "starter," or source of the acid-producing bacteria.

MOTHER OF VINEGAR

If you see a jellylike cloudy film collecting in the bottom of your vinegar bottle, you've discovered the "mother of vinegar." It's merely cellulose made by acid-producing bacteria. Mother of vinegar is a completely natural by-product of vinegar that contains live bacteria. It is harmless and is not a sign of contamination. Just strain off the liquid vinegar and continue using it.

Most manufacturers pasteurize their vinegar to prevent mother of vinegar from forming. Some say this goo prevents infectious diseases if you eat a little each day, but there is no research to verify that belief.

- Keep the liquid between 60 degrees and 80 degrees Fahrenheit during the fermentation process; it will take three to four weeks to make vinegar. If you keep the liquid too cool, the vinegar may be unusable. If it's kept too warm, it may not form the mother of vinegar mat at the bottom of the container. The mother of vinegar mat signifies proper fermentation.

- Stir the liquid daily to introduce adequate amounts of oxygen, which is necessary for fermentation.

- After three to four weeks, the bacteria will have converted most of the alcohol, and the mixture will begin to smell like vinegar. Taste a little bit each day until it reaches a flavor and acidity that you like.

- Strain the liquid through a cheesecloth or coffee filter several times to remove the mother of vinegar. Otherwise the fermentation process will continue and eventually spoil your vinegar.

- Store in sterilized, capped jars in the refrigerator.

- If you want to store homemade vinegar at room temperature for more than a few months, you must pasteurize it. Do this by heating it to 170 degrees Fahrenheit (use a cooking thermometer to determine the temperature) and hold it at this temperature for 10 minutes. Put the pasteurized vinegar in sterilized containers with tight-fitting lids, out of direct sunlight.

NATURAL CLEANING

Rather than use harsh chemical products for cleaning, see what vinegar can do for you! Note that for cleaning, distilled white vinegar is generally the best choice.

For **everyday cleaning of tile and grout**, rub with a little apple cider vinegar on a sponge. This gives off a pleasant scent and will help cut any greasy buildup.

Mix equal amounts of white vinegar and water in a spray bottle. Spray onto **mildewed areas** and let sit for 15 minutes. Wipe clean. Use as a preventive measure in any area of your home that is prone to being damp, such as spaces under a sink or in the cellar.

Clean marble with a paste of baking soda and distilled white vinegar. Wipe clean and buff.

A **bathtub ring** requires a strong solvent. Try soaking paper towels with undiluted vinegar and placing them on the ring. Let towels dry out, then spray the tub with straight vinegar and scrub with a sponge.

Loosen up **soap scum** on shower doors and walls by spraying them with apple cider or white vinegar. Let dry, then respray to dampen. Wipe clean. Reapply and let sit for several hours. Then dampen and wipe clean again.

Shower curtains can become dulled by soap film or plagued with mildew. Keep vinegar in a spray bottle near your shower, and squirt shower curtains once or twice a week. No need to rinse.

For routine cleaning of **sink and tub drains**, pour in 1/2 cup baking soda followed by 1 cup distilled white vinegar. Let sit for 10 to 20 minutes, then flush with very hot water.

PET CARE

After a therapeutic shampoo to treat a **skin infection,** rinse dog with a solution of 1 part apple cider vinegar to 3 parts water.

Floppy-eared dogs can be prone to **yeast infections in their ears,** especially after bathing or grooming. To avoid getting water in your dog's ears, plug them with cotton balls moistened with diluted apple cider vinegar.

Add 1 tablespoon apple cider vinegar to your pet's water bowl to improve **overall health and digestion.**

An apple a day keeps the flies away: Pour 1/4 cup apple cider vinegar onto a horse's regular grain feed once a day to **deter flies.**

VINEGAR STORAGE

Storing vinegar properly will hold flavor at its peak. Due to their high acid content, commercially prepared vinegars will keep almost indefinitely, even at room temperature. White vinegar will maintain its color, but other kinds may develop an off color or a haze. Neither of these conditions is a sign of spoilage; the vinegar is still good to use.

Store all vinegars in bottles sealed with airtight lids. Keep in a dark, cool place, and avoid direct sunlight, which can diminish flavor, color, and acidity. Homemade vinegars, especially herbal ones, are best stored in the refrigerator.

VITAL VINEGAR

Much more research needs to be done to investigate all of vinegar's healing potential. But even with the evidence available, it's clear that vinegar holds some healing powers. It is not a too-good-to-be-true miracle cure, but it can be used in a variety of ways to enhance your efforts to fight even serious, chronic diseases.

In that sense, vinegar is like many of the other lifestyle adjustments, drugs, and therapies used in our battles against common, chronic, and often life-threatening diseases: It is just one of a variety of important steps that can help us defend ourselves. But unlike many of the other elements that go into treating or preventing disease, vinegar is one you'll certainly enjoy incorporating into your kitchen, your diet, and your life!